YOUR KNOWLEDGE HAS VALUE

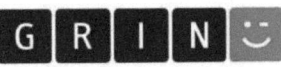

Major Snail Borne Trematode Infections in Cattle

Isayas Asefa

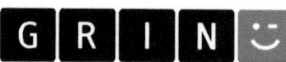

Bibliographic information published by the German National Library:

The German National Library lists this publication in the National Bibliography; detailed bibliographic data are available on the Internet at http://dnb.dnb.de.

ISBN: 9783346662835
This book is also available as an ebook.

© GRIN Publishing GmbH
Nymphenburger Straße 86
80636 München

Print and binding: Books on Demand GmbH, Norderstedt, Germany
Printed on acid-free paper from responsible sources.

The present work has been carefully prepared. Nevertheless, authors and publishers do not incur liability for the correctness of information, notes, links and advice as well as any printing errors.

GRIN web shop: https://www.grin.com/document/1192280

MAJOR SNAIL BORNE TREMATODE INFECTIONS CATTLE: REVIEW

Isayas Asefa

School of Veterinary Medicine, Wolaita Sodo University, P.O. Box 138, Wolaita Sodo, Ethiopia.

Abstract

Snail-borne parasitic sicknesses, for example, fascioliasis, paragonimiasis and schistosomiasis, present dangers to human wellbeing and create major financial issues in numerous tropical and sub-tropical nations. In this survey we sum up the center jobs of snails in the existence patterns of the parasites they have, their clinical indications and sickness disseminations, just as snail control strategies. Snails play four parts in the existence patterns of the parasites they have: as a middle of the road have contaminated by the principal stage hatchlings, as the main halfway host tainted by miracidia, as the primary moderate host that ingests the parasite eggs are ingested, and as the main transitional host entered by miracidia with or without the subsequent middle of the road have been an oceanic creature. Snail-borne parasitic infections target numerous organs, like the lungs, liver, biliary parcel, digestion tracts, mind and kidneys, prompting overactive resistant reactions, diseases, organ disappointment, barrenness and even demise. Non-industrial nations in Africa, Asia and Latin America have the most noteworthy occurrences of these infections, while a few endemic parasites have formed into overall pestilences through the worldwide spread of snails. Physical, synthetic and natural techniques have been acquainted with control the host snail populaces to forestall infection.

Keywords: fascioliasis; Paramphistomes; schistosomiasis

Contents

1. INTRODUCTION

Ethiopia has the largest domesticated animals crowd in sub-Saharan Africa, with an expected cattle populace of 52 million, sheep populace of 25.5 million, and goat populace of almost 24 million. Cattles are the most financially significant animals species with high assessed populace and the larger parts are native zebu breed. Notwithstanding the presence of tremendous number of ruminant populaces, Ethiopia neglects to ideally take advantage of these assets because of various factors, for example, repetitive dry season, foundations issue, uncontrolled animal infections, helpless nourishment, helpless farming practices, and deficiency of prepared labor and absence of government approaches for disease anticipation and control (Bayou and Geda, 2018).

Parasitic diseases extraordinarily affect dairy cattle efficiency and government assistance in all areas of the world. Diseases with two groups of inside parasites liver flukes and gastrointestinal nematodes are usually viewed as generally negative for cattle (Kowalczyk et al., 2018). Particularly, Parasitic diseases brought about by helminthes, protozoa and arthropods can cause more monetary misfortunes than illness brought about by microbes and infections yet their effect nonetheless, isn't obvious to animal proprietors (Shitaye et al., 2007).

Among parasitic diseases 'Trematode infections', particularly fasciolosis, are probably the most financially significant helminth diseases hampering the efficiency of homegrown ruminants around the world (Dargie, 1987; Mage et al., 2002; Njau et al., 1988). All the trematode species which are parasitic in domesticated animals have a place with the subclass Digenea (Hansen and Perry, 1994). The adult trematodes are regularly called 'flukes' and the families which incorporate parasites of significant veterinary significance are Fasciolidae, Dicrocoeliidae, Paramphistomatidae and Schistosomatidae (Andrews, 1999; Urquhart et al., 1996).

4

Fasciola (liver fluke), Paramphistomes (rumen/stomach fluke) and Schistosoma (blood fluke) are the main flukes recorded from various areas of the planet (Dreyfuss *et al.*, 2006).

Fasciolosis is a financially significant illness of homegrown domesticated animals, specifically cattle and sheep, and incidentally man. Fasciola *hepatica* and F. *gigantica* are the two species most generally embroiled as the etiological agents of fasciolosis (Andrews, 1999). Infection of adult dairy cattle with liver flukes, except if in weighty diseases, is normally clinically in clear. Consequently, under ordinary conditions, clinical infection is just reasonable in youthful cattle (Love, 2017). Be that as it may, even unassuming infection can bring about huge decrease in milk yield and quality (Urquhart *et al.*, 1996), decrease in weight gain (Hope-Cawdery *et al.*, 1977; Ross, 1970) and reproductives execution (Elliott *et al.*, 2015).

Paramphistomes Fischoeder 1901, otherwise called rumen flukes, are gastrointestinal trematodes having a place with the group of Paramphistomatidae (Soulsby, 1982). These are narrowly formed flukes estimating 5–12mm× 2–4 mm. The grown-ups' preference destinations are the rumen and reticulum of ruminants while the juvenile parasites are found in the small digestive organs and stomach (Rojo-Vázquez *et al.*, 2012).

They are to a great extent non-pathogenic however clinical flare-ups have been accounted for to happen. The main species in Africa is Paramphistomum *microbothrium* (Dinnik, 1964). Others are Paramphistomum *cervi* (European Environment Agency, 2004), Paramphistomum *ichikawar* (Australasia) (FAO, 1993) and Paramphistomum *daubneyi* (first depicted in Kenya and normal in Europe) (Abrous *et al.*, 1996). The adult paramphistomes are viewed as commensals in the rumen, as weighty infections are endured without making any harm the rumen (Dinnik, 1964), albeit juvenile parasites in the small digestive system cause clinical disease (Aiello, 1998).

Schistosomosis in dairy cattle in Africa can be brought about by Schistosoma *bovis*, S. *mattheei* and S. *leiperi*. Schistosomosis is for the most part viewed as of low significance in enormous ruminants, and even where a high predominance of the parasite is distinguished in butchered cattle, clinical indications of the infections are seen just once in a long while (Urquhart *et al.*, 1996). Be that as it may, infections here and there might bring about serious clinical signs (Hansen and Perry, 1994).

Despites the meanings of the trematode diseases in veterinary medicine, there are not many examinations about trematode infections in enormous ruminants in most piece of southern Ethiopia. Accordingly, the current review was planned with the accompanying destinations:

➢ To gauge the pervasiveness of trematode infections in cattle and

➢ To distinguishing hazard factors related with disease of cattle with trematodes at Humbo woreda.

2. LITERATURE REVIEW

2.1. Definition and Taxonomy

Helminth parasites falls under two phyla specifically Nemathelminthes (roundworms) and Platyhelminthes (flatworms) Phylum platyhelminths contain the two classes of parasitic level worms, the Trematoda and the Cestoda. The class Trematoda falls into two primary subclasses, the Monogenia which have an immediate life cycle, and the Digenia which require a middle host. There are numerous families in the class Trematoda and those which incorporate parasites of the significant veterinary significance are the Fasciolidae, Dicrocoeliidae, Paramphistomatidae and Schistosomatidae (Urquhart *et al.*, 1996). Of the lesser significance are the Troglotrematidae and Opisthorchiidae.

Adult trematodes (flukes) are typically simple to perceive as a result of their level leaf-like shape and the conspicuous presence of suckers. There are two trematode groups of veterinary interest: those found as ectoparasites on fish (Monogenean trematodes) and those that are endoparasites in vertebrates (digenean trematodes). Monogenean trematodes have a solitary oral sucker in addition to numerous suckers mounted on an unmistakable back connection organ (the haptor). They have direct lifecycles and, as there is no transitional host, diseases can spread quickly by direct transmission in hydroponics systems (Jacobs, 2009)

The Digenea is probably the largest group of platyhelminths and parasitizes a wide scope of invertebrate and vertebrate hosts which additionally incorporates people. Inside the vertebrate, last host, these worms are found in various organs, including the digestive tract, lungs, liver, and vascular system. Diseases with these parasites are liable for significant production misfortunes in the domesticated animals industry and lessening in the personal satisfaction in people (Fürst *et al.*, 2012; Mas-Coma *et al.*, 2005; Piedrafita *et al.*, 2010; Qian *et al.*, 2016; Walz *et al.*, 2015).

Digenean trematodes have only two suckers – ventral and oral. The mouth leads from the last option to a solid pharynx which siphons food into two visually impaired consummation caeca. In certain genera, like Fasciola, these are extended to build surface region. There is no butt, so they need to disgorge squander materials through the mouth. There is an ovary, two testicles and vitelline organs which produce the eggshell. In the liver, Fasciola makes production misfortunes worldwide in ruminants with access wet fields, Dicrocoelium is less harming and found in drier conditions, while Fascioloides is innocuous in wild ruminants yet deadly to sheep. Adult amphistomes are for the most part harmless however their juvenile stages can have extreme and, in some cases, deadly outcomes in hotter, wetter areas. The schistosomes are not kidding microorganisms, generally bound to the jungles. Some happen solely in people, some in animals, while a couple are equipped for move from animals to individuals or visa-versa. (Jacobs, 2009)

2.2. Etiology

2.2.1. Fasciola (Liver Fluke)

The two most significant species are F. *hepatica* and F. *gigantica* (Dubinský, 1993). Fasciola *gigantica* is solely tropical and measures (27 to 75mm) x (3 to 12mm) though, F. *hepatica* is found in calm regions (high elevation districts in east Africa) and measures roughly (20 to 30mm) x (10mm) (Brown, 1980).

2.2.2. Paramphistomes (Rumen/Stomach Fluke)

There are various types of paramphistomes A few significant animal varieties are Paramphistomum *cervi*, Paramphistomum *cotylophorum*, Paramphistomum cracile, Paramphistomum *gotoi*, Paramphistomum *grande*, Paramphistomum *hiberniae*, Paramphistomum *ichikawai*, Paramphistomum *epiclitum*, Paramphistomum *explanatum*, Paramphistomum *leydeni*, Paramphistomum *liorchis*, Paramphistomum *microbothrioides*, Paramphistomum *phillerouxi* (Lotfy *et al.*, 2010).

2.2.3. Schistosoma (Blood Fluke)

Homegrown animals in different tropical regions might be impacted with Schistosoma (S). *bovis*, S. *indicus*, S. *nasalis*, S. *suis*, S. *matheei* (Bowman *et al.*, 2003). Schistosoma japonicum was likewise announced in human, felines and different vertebrates in Africa (Dwight *et al.*, 2003).

2.3. Morphology

Figure 1: Mature schistosome worm: female lying in the gynaecophoric canal of male

Editor's note: This image was removed due to copyright reasons.

Figure 1. The life cycle of *F. hepatica*; the sheep liver fluke (Source: http://www.dpd.cdc, accessed on january22, 2022).

2.4. Life Cycles

2.4.1. Fasciola (Liver Fluke)

Juvenile eggs are released in the biliary conduits and in the stool. Eggs become embryonated in water; eggs discharge miracidia, which attack a reasonable snail halfway host, including the genera Galba, Fossaria and Pseudosuccinea. In the snail the parasites go through a few formative stages (sporocysts, rediae and cercariae). The cercariae are set free from the snail and encyst as metacercariae on oceanic vegetation or different surfaces. Warm blooded animals procure the infection by eating vegetation containing metacercariae. People can become tainted by ingesting metacercariae-containing new water plants, particularly watercress. After ingestion, the metacercariae excyst in the duodenum and relocate through the gastrointestinal divider, the peritoneal pit and the liver parenchyma into the biliary conduits, where they form into adults (http://www.dpd.cdc, 2022 and Urquhart *et al.*, 1996).

2.4.2. Paramphistomes (Rumen/Stomach Fluke)

The rumen fluke life cycle requires two hosts including snail moderate and mammalians generally ruminants conclusive host. The infection of the definitive host is started by the ingestion of encysted metacercariae joined to vegetation or drifting in water (González *et al.*, 2013). Their life cycle is aberrant, requiring conclusive has, for example, a ruminant and a middle host like a snail. The physically adult monoecious self-treated in the mammalian rumen and delivery the egg alongside the excrement. Egg hatch in water into ciliated miracidia. The miracidia then enter the body of a moderate host which is snails having a place with genera Bulinus, Planorbis and stagnicola (Bowman, 2008).

Adult flukes in the stomach lay eggs that are shed outside with the feces. Around fourteen days after the fact miracidia hatch out of the eggs. They swim in the water until they track down a reasonable snail. They enter the snail and proceed with advancement to sporocysts and rediae, which can increase asexually and produce little daughter rediae. Every media contains around 15-30 cercariae. Mature cercariae are moved by two eyespots and a long slim tail, by which they track down amphibian plants or other appropriate foundations to which they get joined and encyst to become metacercariae (Jones *et al.*, 2017).

The mammalian hosts ingest the infective larvae. Once inside the duodenum and jejunum, their cysts are in eliminated (Arrue *et al.*, 1970). They enter the gastrointestinal divider by effectively annihilating the mucosa and afterward relocate to the rumen, where they complete improvement to adult flukes and begin creating eggs. After ingestion by the last host, it requires 2 to 4 months for metacercariae to finish improvement and begin laying eggs (pre-patent period) (Sanabria and Romero, 2008).

2.4.3. Schistosoma (Blood Fluke)

Schistosomes have a commonplace trematode vertebrate invertebrate lifecycle (Laurant, 2013). Schistosomes live in the mesenteric and hepatic veins of the host (aside from S. *nasale*, which lives in the nasal veins), where they feed on blood and produce eggs with a trademark terminal or sidelong spine (Merck and Dhome, 2010).

Parasite eggs are set into the climate free from tainted individuals, bring forth on contact with new water to deliver the free-swimming miracidium. Miracidia contaminate

10

freshwater snails by infiltrating the snail's foot. After disease, near the site of infiltration, the miracidium changes into an essential (mother) sporocyst (Laurant, 2013). Microorganism cells inside the essential sporocyst will then, at that point, start separating to deliver auxiliary (daughter) sporocysts, which relocate to the snail's hepatopancreas. Once at the hepatopancreas, microbe cells inside the auxiliary sporocyst start to partition once more, this time creating huge number of new parasites, known as cercariae, which are the larvae fit for contaminating vertebrates (Laurant, 2013).

Cercariae arise every day from the snail have in a circadian musicality, reliant upon surrounding temperature and light. Youthful cercariae are profoundly versatile, switching back and forth between energetic vertical developments and sinking to keep up with their situation in the water. Cercarial movement is especially invigorated by water disturbance, by shadows and by synthetic compounds found on human skin (Fenwick, 2012).

Editor's note: This image was removed due to copyright reasons.
Figure 2: Life cycle of Schistosomes; Source: (CDC, 2011)

2.5. Epidemiology

2.5.1. *Fasciola (Liver* Fluke*)*

Geographic Distribution:

Human and animal fasciolosis happen around the world (Torgerson and Claxton, 1999). While animal fasciolosis is appropriated in nations with high cattle and sheep production, human fasciolosis happens, aside from Western Europe, in emerging nations. Fasciolosis happens just in regions where appropriate conditions for middle of the host has exist (Torgerson and Claxton, 1999)

Environment of Intermediate Host:

The Lymnae *truncatula* is the vastest spread and significant species developed in the transmission of F. *hepatica*. The snails are land and/or water capable and despite the fact that they go through hours in shallow water, they occasionally arise on to the encompassing mud. They are equipped for enduring summer dry season or winter freezing for a long time by individually aestivating and sleeping somewhere down in the mud. Ideal conditions incorporate a marginally corrosive pH climate and a gradually moving water medium to divert byproducts. They feed generally on green growth and the ideal temperature range for improvement is 15 to 22 °C; under 5 °C advancement stops (Urquhart *et al.*, 1996). This snail is usually seen in ineffectively depleted land, waste trenches and areas of leakages of spring or broken channels, sloppy passages, vehicle wheel grooves, wet and sloppy spots close to drinking box and foot prints of animals on mud soil (Soulsby, 1968).

Factors Influencing the Agent:

The primary variables deciding the circumstance and seriousness of metacercariae collecting on herbage are recorded underneath. Specifically, temperature and dampness (precipitation) influence both spatial and worldly plenitude of snail have and the pace of advancement of fluke egg and larvae. Four principal factors vital for the flare-up of fasciolosis impacting the production of metacercariae are: the accessibility of reasonable snail and its propensity, temperature, dampness and pH (Radostits *et al.*, 2007; Urquhart *et al.*, 1996).

Accessibility of reasonable snail and its propensity:

Lymnae *truncatula* lean towards wet mud to free water and extremely durable natural surroundings incorporates the banks of trenches or streams and the edges of little lakes, following weighty precipitation or flooding, brief territories might be given by foot marks, wheel grooves, or downpour lakes. However marginally corrosive pH climate is ideal for Lymnae *truncatula*, unnecessarily corrosive pH levels are adverse (Radostits *et al.*, 2007; Urquhart *et al.*, 1996; Rowcliff and Ollerenshow, 1960)

Temperature:

Temperature is a significant variable influencing the advancement pace of snails and the phases of parasites outside the host. The mean constantly temperature of 10 °C or above is important for the snail host to raise and for the F. *hepatica* to create inside the snail (Radostits *et al*., 2007). Movements of every kind stop at temperature underneath 5 °C. This is additionally least reach for the turn of events and incubating of F. *hepatica* eggs. Nonetheless, it is just when temperature ascends to 15 °C and is kept up with over this level that a huge increase of snails and fluke larvae stages guarantees (Urquhart *et al*., 1996).

Dampness:

The ideal dampness condition for snail rearing and the advancement of F. *hepatica* inside snails are given when precipitation surpasses happening and field immersion is achieved. Such conditions are likewise fundamental for the improvement of fluke eggs, for miracidia looking for snails and for the dispersal of cercariae being shed from the snail (Urquhart *et al*., 1996)

pH:

Fields with bunches of surges are normal locales having a slight pH. Eggs brooded at 27 °C will create and bring forth inside a pH scope of 4.2 to 9.0, however improvement is drawn out when pH surpasses 8.0 (Rowcliff and Ollerenshow, 1960).

2.5.2. Paramphistomes (Rumen/Stomach Fluke)

Paramphistomum is appropriated from one side of the planet to the other, yet the most noteworthy commonness has been in tropical and subtropical locales, especially in Africa, Asia, Australia, Eastern Europe and Russia (Rolfe *et al*., 1994). The study of disease transmission of Paramphistomosis controlled by a few elements administered by parasite-have climate communications. The major epidemiological variable impacting the worm weights of animals is the disease rate from pastures. It is likewise impacted by the climatic necessity for egg bring forth, advancement and endurance in field (Ozdal *et al.*, 2010).

In Ethiopia, Paramphistomosis has been accounted for from various pieces of the country with roughly 45.83%in western Gojam, 28.6% in Debrezeit and 6.7% in Hawassa and there is a shortage of very much reported data on the event of paramphistomum in ruminants in brushing around Lake Ashenge (Tsegabirhan *et al.*, 2015).

2.5.3. Schistosoma (Blood Fluke)

It is practically like Fasciola *gigantica* and Paramphistomes. Schistosoma required water for incubating of the eggs. Eggs can incubate in somewhat acidic pH. Shedding of cercariae is temperature subordinate. Long time is needed for improvement of Schistosoma in snail high downpour fall is great inclining factor for event of these parasites (Mandal, 2012). Epidemiological examinations on Bovine schistosomiasis are reminiscent of the endemicity of the illness especially in regions with enormous extremely durable water bodies and muddy field regions. In Ethiopia, the ideal reach for conveyance of S. *mansoni* has been accounted for as 1500 to 2000 meter above ocean level (m.a.s.l) (Gashaw, 2010).

2.6. Host Range

2.6.1. Definitive Host

Fasciola (Liver Fluke):

The last host are sheep, goats, cattle, horse, deer, man and different warm-blooded animals in which its standard site is the liver (Taylor, 2007). The adolescent stage moves and became developed inside the biliary arrangement of the liver. At the point when the specialist becomes adult, it plugs the conduit system. The adult one gives egg that is delivered with bile emission in to destroy where it was discharged with excrement (Urquhart *et al.*, 1996).

Paramphistomes (Rumen/Stomach Fluke):

Paramphistomum contaminates cattle, sheep, goats and other domesticated animals just as numerous wild ruminants. Ruminants are authoritative hosts (González *et al.*, 2013).

Schistosoma (Blood Fluke):

Every single homegrown warm-blooded animal. Fundamentally significant in sheep and dairy cattle (Urquhart *et al.*, 1996).

2.6.2. Transitional Host

Fasciola (Liver Fluke):

Galba *truncatula*, the most widely recognized moderate host of F. *hepatica* in Europe and South America. Moderate hosts of F. *hepatica* are freshwater snails from family Lymnaeidae (Torgerson and Claxton, 1999; Graczyk *et al.*, 1999). Snails from family Planorbidae go about as a middle host of F. *hepatica* sporadically (Mas-Coma *et al.*, 2005). Coming up next are significant species associated with the transmission of F. *hepatica* and are liable for the improvement of miracidium to cercaria phases of Fasciola larvae (Smyth, 1994).

Table 1: Snail intermediate host and their distribution

Snail intermediate host	Country
Lymnae *truncatula*	Europe
Lymnae stagnalis	Europe
Lymnae viator	Peru
Lymnae columella	New Zealand
Lymnae tomentosa	Australia
Lymnae natalensis	West and Eastern Africa

Lymnae rufescens	West Africa
Lymnae glarba	Europe

Figure 4. Shell layers of Galba *truncatula*; intermediate host of Fasciola *hepatica*

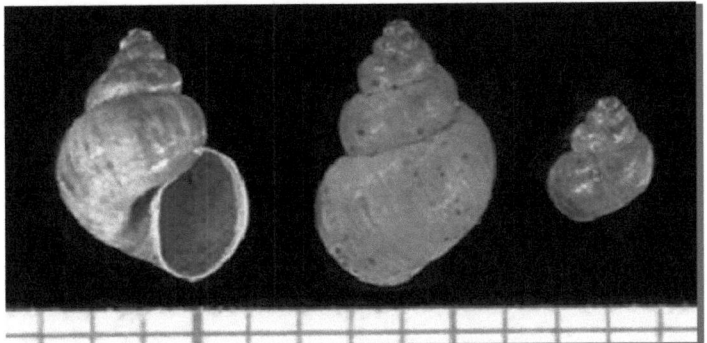

(Source: Torgerson and Claxton, 1999).

Paramphistomes (Rumen/Stomach Fluke):

Freshwater snail goes about as the transitional host of the variety Bulinus, Planorbis, Stagnicola (Tsegabirhan *et al.*, 2015).

Schistosoma (Blood Fluke):

Water snails like Bulinus and Physopsis spp. curve especially significant in the transmission of cow-like and ovine schistosomiasis ((Urquhart *et al.*, 1996).

2.7. Pathogenesis

2.7.1. Fasciola (Liver Fluke)

The advancement of disease in definitive host is separated into two stages which are the parenchymal (transitory) stage and the biliary stage (Dubinský, 1993). The parenchymal stage starts when excysted adolescent flukes infiltrate the digestive divider. After the infiltration of the digestive tract, flukes move inside the stomach hole and enter the liver or different organs. F. *hepatica* has a solid inclination for the tissues of the liver (Behm and Sangster, 1999). Sporadically, ectopic areas of flukes like the lungs, stomach, digestive divider, kidneys, and subcutaneous tissue can happen (Chen and Mott, 1990; Boray, 1969). During the movement of flukes, tissues are precisely annihilated and aggravation shows up around transitory tracks of flukes. The subsequent stage (the biliary stage) starts when parasites enter the biliary conduits of the liver. In biliary conduits, flukes mature, feed on blood, and produce eggs. Hypertrophy of biliary conduits related with obstacle of the lumen happens because of tissue harm (Taylor, 2007; Urquhart *et al.*, 1996).

2.7.2. Paramphistomes (Rumen/Stomach Fluke)

The pathogenesis impact of rumen fluke is related with the gastrointestinal period of infection. The youthful fluke is plug feeders and this outcomes in extreme disintegration of the duodenal mucosa. In weighty infection, this reason enteritis described by edema, discharge and ulceration (Dube and Aisien, 2010). In tropical districts this Paramphistomosis has been viewed as an exceptionally pathogenic disease , it causes enteritis and paleness in domesticated animals well evolved animals and result in considerable production and monetary misfortunes (Dorny *et al.*, 2011).

Neurotic manifestations are created by juvenile flukes. At the point when the youthful flukes begin to assemble in digestive system, there is watery and rank the runs which is regularly connected with high mortality (even up to 80-90%). In ruminants, at a given time upwards of 30, 000 flukes might gather, intensely assaulting the duodenal mucosa to initiate intense enteritis. Adult flukes are somewhat innocuous and liver tissue is for the most part harmed widely shown by enlarging, drain, staining, putrefaction, bile conduit hyperplasia and fibrosis (Bilqees *et al.*, 211). In weighty infection of beforehand uninfected youthful animals, the juvenile helminths connect to the duodenal mucosa utilizing their power full ventral sucker and profoundly implanted in the mucosa causing serious enteritis, duodenitis, hypoproteinemia, edema, drain and potentially corruption.

17

The neurotic sore leads animals to show anorexia, polydipsia, serious looseness of the bowels and demise due to juvenile paramphistomum is exceptionally high and perhaps as high as 80% to 90% in homegrown ruminants (Juyal et al., 2003).

The ruminal sore has additionally been related with weighty disease by the adult worm of paramphistomum ichikawai (Rolfe et al, 1994) and C. microbothrium which might have impacted processing and assimilation bringing about the runs, anorexia, iron deficiency and shortcoming (Dorny et al., 2011). P. cerviare plug feeders and cause genuine infection by covering themselves into the submucosa of the duodenum and benefiting from epithelial cells of the burners organ bringing about anorexia, perfuse foul looseness of the bowels drop in plasma protein's focus and sickliness which debilitates the host (Dube and Aisien, 2010.).

2.7.3. Schistosoma (Blood Fluke)

Schistosomiasis (or bilharziasis) is surprising among helminth infections for two reasons: a large part of the pathogenesis is because of the eggs (rather than larvae or grown-ups); and the vast majority of the pathology is brought about by have insusceptible reactions (deferred type extreme touchiness and granulomatous responses) (Oliveira et al., 2004). The course of disease is frequently partitioned into three stages: transient, intense and ongoing. The transient stage happens when cercariae infiltrate and relocate through the skin. This is regularly asymptomatic, yet in sharpened patients, it might cause transient dermatitis ('swimmers tingle'), and at times aspiratory injuries and pneumonitis (Oliveira et al., 2004).

Eggs delivered into the circulation system by adult worms can attack neighborhood tissues, where they discharge poisons and compounds and incite a TH-2-interceded insusceptible reaction (Coutinho et al., 2007). Aggravation and granuloma development happens around saved eggs, which can prompt fibrosis and scarring of impacted tissues, on the off chance that the weight of eggs is weighty (Cheever et al., 2000). Eggs will

18

more often than not either enter the inside (neighboring the mesenteric vessels where the adult worms are living) or travel by means of the entry venous system to the liver. In the inside, granulomatous irritation around the attacking eggs can bring about digestive schistosomiasis portrayed by ulceration and scarring (Friedman et al., 2007).

The movement of the eggs might cause mechanical harm and sores. Besides, Schistosoma eggs caught in the tissue inspire granulomatous response that is mounted to destruct the eggs. These granulomas comprise of a few cell types, essentially eosinophils, macrophages and lymphocytes. In the constant phases of the illness the pathology is related with collagen testimony and fibrosis, bringing about organ harm and brokenness (Koqulan and Lucely, 2005).

2.8. Clinical sign

2.8.1. Fasciola (Liver Fluke)

Clinical indications of fasciolosis are firmly related 100% of the time with infection dose(measure of ingested metacercariae). Fusciola diseases might cause a deficiency of production in draining cattle during winter. Clinically, these are hard to distinguish since the fluke burdens are typically low and pallor isn't clear. The primary impacts circular segment a decrease in milk yield and quality, especially of the solids-not-fat part. In cattle and sheep, as the most well-known conclusive host, clinical show is separated into 4 kinds (Radostits et al., 2007; Behm and Sangster, 1999; Urquhart et al., 1996 and Dubinský, 1993). The four clinical sorts of fasciolosis might be show up:

I) Acute Type I Fasciolosis: infection dose is more than 5000 ingested metacercariae. animals abruptly bite the dust with next to no past clinical signs. Ascites, stomach discharge, icterus, paleness of layers, shortcoming might be noticed (Radostits et al., 2007; Behm and Sangster, 1999).

ii) Acute Type II Fasciolosis: infection dose is 1000-5000 ingested metacercariae. As above, may prompt passing however momentarily show paleness, loss of condition and ascites (Urquhart *et al* 1996).

iii) Sub intense Fasciolosis: infection dose is 800-1000 ingested metacercariae. Sheep and cattle are lazy, iron deficient and may bite the dust. Weight reduction is a predominant aspect (Radostits *et al.*, 2007 and Urquhart *et al.*, 1996).

iv) Chronic Fasciolosis: infection dose is 200-800 ingested metacercariae. Asymptomatic or slow improvement of container jaw and ascites (ventral edema), anorexia, weight reduction, iron deficiency, hypo-albuminemia and eosinophilia might be seen in a wide range of fasciolosis (Behm and Sangster, 1999; Dubinský, 1993).

2.8.2. Paramphistomes (Rumen/Stomach Fluke)

Rumen fluke which is for the most part parasitizing domesticated animals ruminants, just as a few wild well evolved animals are liable for the genuine disease called Paramphistomosis otherwise called amphistomosis particularly in cattle and sheep. Its manifestations incorporate plentiful loose bowels, frailty, dormancy and frequently bring about death if untreated. The major clinical indication of stomach fluke infection is enteritis (irritation of the small digestive tract) and solid the runs (watery scour) with blood follows as a result parchedness, bluntness, weight reduction, and so forth Iron deficiency and jug jaw can likewise create (Olsen, 1974).

Juvenile rumen fluke is a fitting feeder (Melaku. what's more Addis, 2012.) and causes genuine infection by covering themselves into the submucosa of the duodenum and benefiting from the epithelial cells of the Brunner's organ bringing about anorexia perfuse offensive the runs, drop in plasma protein focus and paleness, which debilitates the host. Mature paramphistomum is additionally answerable for sporadic rumination, rumenitis, lower nourishing change and loss of body condition, anorexia, polydipsia and serious the runs (Olsen, 1974).

20

2.8.3. Schistosoma (Blood Fluke)

In cattle the clinical sign showed anorexia checked the runs, blended in with blood or mucous, drying out pale of mucous film, stamped weight reduction, diminished production, harsh hair coat, weakness, hypoalbuminemia, hyperglobulinemia and serious eosinophilia that create after the beginning of egg discharge. Seriously impacted animals fall apart quickly and typically bite the dust inside a couple of long stretches of infection, while those less intensely tainted fosters constant illness with development impediment (Merck and Dhome, 2010).

Hemorrhagic enteritis, paleness and starvation which create after the beginning of eggs discharge, are major clinical signs related with the digestive and hepatic structure schistosomiasis in ruminants seriously impacted animals disintegrate quickly and as a rule bite the dust inside a couple of long periods of infection (Charles and Robinson, 2004).

9. Finding and Diagnosis

2.9.1. Fasciola (Liver Fluke)

Finding depends overwhelmingly on feces assessments and immunological strategies. In any case, clinical signs, biochemical and hematological profile, season, environment conditions, the study of disease transmission circumstance, and assessments of snails should be thought of (Torgerson and Claxton, 1999; Dubinský, 1993). In light of this data, various strategies are utilized to analyze the infection like fluke egg count, liver compound location, after death assessment (Urquhart *et al.*, 1996).

After death Examination:

Assessment of new corpses is the best technique for determination on the off chance that liver fluke is suspected. As untreated animals give the most dependable sign of the liver

21

fluke and times of challenge, posthumous assessment will likewise show any sores coming about because of simultaneous illness like dark infection or parasitic gastro enteritis (Urquhart *et al.*, 1996). There is no fix and passing follows rapidly. As Clostridium novyi is normal in the climate, dark illness is found any place populaces of liver flukes and sheep cross-over. Despite the fact that, it is difficult to recognize Fasciola in live animals, liver assessment at butcher or necropsy was viewed as the most immediate, solid and financially savvy procedure for the analysis of Fasciolosis (Urquhart *et al.*, 1996).

Fluke Egg Count:

Conclusion of fasciola is affirmed by tracking down the eggs in the excrement. These eggs should be recognized from the eggs of different flukes particularly the enormous eggs of paramphistomes (Soulsby, 1968). The Fasciola eggs are oval, yellow brown and measures (130 to 150μm by 60 to 90 μm). Each egg will have a particular operculum (Hendrix and Robinson, 2007).

Serological Detection:

Different serological procedures on blood tests including ELISA can be utilized to identify antibodies of Fasciola *hepatica* with undeniable degree of explicitness (Urquhart *et al.*, 1996). Antibodies against parts of flukes are recognized in serum or milk tests, the ELISA and latent trim agglutination test, being the most solid (Taylor, 2007).

Recognizing Liver Enzymes:

Two proteins are normally estimated, glutamate dehydrogenase (GLDH), is delivered when parenchymal cells are harmed and levels become raised inside the initial not many long stretches of disease. The other gamma-glutamyl transferase (GGT) demonstrates harm of epithelial cells coating the bile pipes and raised levels are kept up with for longer periods (Taylor, 2007). Height of liver compound exercises, such a glutamate dehydrogenase (GLDH), gamma-glutamyl transferase (GGT), and lactate dehydrogenase

(LDH), is distinguished in subacute or ongoing fasciolosis from 12-multi week after ingestion of metacercariae (Anderson *et al.*, 1981; Sykes *et al.*, 1980).

2.9.2. Paramphistomes (Rumen/Stomach Fluke)

Determination of rumen fluke depends on the clinical sign normally including youthful animals in the group and history of touching area around the snail environment. Waste example assessment is of little worth since the illness happening during the prepatent period. The affirmation can be acquired by an after-death assessment and recuperation of the little fluke from the duodenum (Urquhart *et al.*, 1996). Side effects are generally noticeable on the conduct of the host. Contaminated sheep and cattle become seriously anorexic or overview food wastefully and become unthrifty. Constant looseness of the bowels is an undeniable sign of weighty infection in the stomach related system, hence an essential finding. The liquid *feces* are analyzed to recognize youthful flukes (Olsen, 1974).

2.9.3. Schistosoma (Blood Fluke)

Assessment of stool or potentially pee for ova is the essential techniques for finding for suspected schistosome infections. The decision of test to analyze schistosomiasis relies upon the types of parasite probably causing the disease. Adult phases of S. mansoni, S. japonicum, S. mekongi, and S. intercalatumreside in the mesenteric venous plexus of contaminated has and eggs are shed in defecation; S. haematobiumadult worms are found in the venous plexus of the lower urinary parcel and eggs are shed in pee (CDC, 2012).

As a general rule, when schistosomiasis is suspected, conclusion is best affirmed by itemized posthumous assessment, which uncover sore and assuming mesentery is extended the presentence of run of the mill injury in the skin that interact with lake, lake, and stream or sea water containing infective cercaria from the snail middle hosts. Waste assessment is generally helpful in early disease, since egg production   decrease as

23

infection advances. Eggs don't have an operculum and most are spindling molded (Bowman *et al.*, 2003).

2.10. Treatment

2.10.1. Fasciola (Liver Fluke)

Various medicine s has been utilized in charge fasciolosis in animals. Drugs contrast in their viability, method of activity, cost, and substance name, business trademark and accessibility available. As indicated by Fairweather and Boray (1999), the Fasciolicides (drugs against Fasciola species) fall into five principal substance bunches as:

A. Halogenated phenols: bithionol (Bitin), hexachlorophene (Bilevon), nitroxynil (Trodax).

B. Salicylanilides: closantel (Flukiver, Supaverm), rafoxanide (Flukanide, Ranizole).

C. Benzimidazoles bunch: triclabendazole (Fasinex), albendazole (Vermitan, Valbazen), mebendazol (Telmin), luxabendazole (Fluxacur)

D. Sulphonamides: clorsulon (Ivomec).

E. Phenoxyalkanes: diamphenetide (Coriban) Triclabendazole (Fasinex) is considered as the most widely recognized medicine because of its high viability against adult just as adolescent flukes.

By and large, Triclabendazole is utilized in charge of fasciolosis of domesticated animals in numerous nations. All things considered, it drawn out veterinary, it made appearance of opposition F. *hepatica*. In animals, its opposition was first depicted in Australia (Overend and Bowen, 1995), later in Ireland (O'Brien, 1998) and Scotland (Mitchell *et al.*, 1998) and all the more as of late in the Netherlands (Moll *et al.*, 2000). Considering this reality, researchers have begun to chip away at the improvement of new medicine. As of late, another Fasciolicide was effectively tried in normally and tentatively contaminated cattle in Mexico. This new medicine is called 'Compound Alpha' and is synthetically basically the same as triclabendazole (Ibarra *et al.*, 2004).

2.10.2. Paramphistomes (Rumen/Stomach Fluke)

Drugs demonstrated to be successful for treatment are resorantel, oxyclozanide, clorsulon, ivermectin, niclosamide, bithional and levamisole (Bowman, 2008).

2.10.3. Schistosoma (Blood Fluke)

Infections with all significant Schistosoma species can be treated with praziquantel. The circumstance of treatment is significant since praziquantel is best against the adult worm and requires the presence of an adult neutralizer reaction to the parasite (CDC, 2012). Throughout the long term, various medicine s with known schistosomocidal yet additionally harmful impacts, for example, antimonials, trichlorphon or nequvon have been tried against instinctive Schistosoma infection in cattle (Reinecke, 1997).

2.11. Control

Fasciola: Control of fasciolosis might be drawn nearer in various ways (Urquhart *et al.*, 1996):

1. Decrease of Snail Population: An overview of the area for snail environments ought to be made to decide if these limited or wide spread. The best long-haul strategy for lessening mud snail populace, for example, Lymnae *truncatula* is seepage since it guarantees super durable obliteration of snail territories. At the point when snail natural surroundings are restricted, a basic technique for control is to fence off this area or treat every year with a molluscicide (CuSO4) (Taylor *et al.*, 2007 and Urquhart *et al.*, 1996). At the point when middle snail have is sea-going, for example, Lymnae *tomentosa*, great control is conceivable by adding a molluscicide to the water territories of the snail (Urquhart *et al.*, 1996).

2. *Anthelmintic Therapy:* The prophylactic utilization of fluke anthelminthics is pointed toward lessening field pollution by fluke eggs all at once generally appropriate for their advancement which goes from April to August in jungles. The eliminating fluke populace during a period of significant weight or at a time of wholesome and pregnancy stress to the animal are another treatment techniques. To accomplish these objectives, the legitimate controlling project is suggested for quite a long time with typical or sub optimal precipitation. Since the hour of treatment depends on the way that most metacercareae show up in pre-winter and late-fall, it might require change for use in different regions (Thomas, 1983). The exact planning of the spring and harvest time treatment will rely upon lambing and administration dates (Urquhart *et al.*, 1996).

3. *Gussing the Occurrence:* The existence pattern of liver flukes and the predominance of fasciolosis is reliant upon environment. This has prompted the improvement of anticipating systems dependent on meteorological information which assesses the reasonable planning and seriousness of the illness. The figure is utilized to give an early admonition of disease by ascertaining information from May to August, so that control measures can be acquainted earlier with shedding of cercareae (Taylor, 2007). Albeit this method is fundamentally applied to summer disease of snail, it is likewise utilized for estimating the colder time of year infection of snail by summating the incentive for August, September and October. The other strategy utilized is 'a wet day' conjecture. This looks at the predominance of Fasciolosis over various years with the quantity of downpour days throughout the late spring of these years. Generally, wide spread fasciolosis is related with 12 wet days (over 1.0mm of precipitation) each month from June to September where temperature don't fall underneath the occasional ordinary (Urquhart *et al.*, 1996).

4. *Immunological Approach:* Antibody is delivered by the host against the antigen in the exsheathing liquid and against proteins made by the worm. Invulnerability could be created by immunizing with antigen material got from helminthes. Helminthes insusceptibility is typically not so much proficient but rather more transient than the invulnerability to microorganisms since, they don't replicate in the host as do microbes, infection and protozoa. Despite the fact that cattle foster a solid resistant response to Fasciola *hepatica* than sheep, the extreme response in cattle brings about hepatic fibrosis, hyperplasia and calcification of the bile channels (Radostits *et al.*, 1994)

Paramphistomes (Rumen/Stomach Fluke):

As in Fasciola the best control is accomplished by giving a funneled water supply to box and forestalling access of the animals to regular water. That being said snails might get close enough to water tanks and standard utilization of a molluscicide at source or manual expulsion of snails might be fundamental (Urquhart et al., 1996).

Schistosoma (Blood Fluke):

This is like that laid out for F gigantica and Paramphistomurn infections. The best method for controlling cattle schistosomiasis in endemic regions is to forestall contact between the animals and the parasite by fencing of hazardous waters and providing clean water. Sadly, this isn't dependably imaginable in areas of the planet where migrant states of the board win. Different techniques for control incorporate annihilation of the snail transitional host populace at transmission locales, either by synthetic or organic strategies, or their expulsion by mechanical boundaries or snail traps (Merck and Dohme, 2010).

In people, the best method of controlling Schistosomosis are the arrangement of sterile offices and the arrangement of funneled water since, it decreases human contact with tainted water (Mohammad and Waqtola, 2006).

2.12. General Health Importance

Fasciola: Studies completed lately have demonstrated human fasciolosis to be a significant general medical issue (Chen and Mott, 1990). Human F. *hepatica* infection is dictated by the presence of the moderate snail has, homegrown herbivorous animals, climatic conditions and the dietary propensities for man (Radostits et al., 2007; Chen and Mott, 1990). Since F. *hepatica* cercariae additionally encyst on water surface, people can be contaminated by drinking of new untreated water containing metacercariae (Chen and Mott, 1990). Moreover, an exploratory review recommended that people burning-through crude liver dishes from new liver tainted with adolescent flukes could become contaminated (Taira et al., 1997).

27

Schistosomiasis, still frequently called the old name of bilharziasis, is of significant significance and along with ancylostomiasis and filariosis circular segment the main helminth diseases of man. The two most normal gastrointestinal species are S. mansoni and S japonicum, the last option once in a while happening in homegrown animals. The third, S. huematohium, is found in the veins of the bladder. A type of cutaneous lama migrans, frequently called 'swimmers tingle'. happens in man and is believed to be brought about by cercariae of avian and animal schistosomes which have a restricted movement in human skin (Urquhart *et al* 1996).

3. REFERENCE

Abrous, M., Rondelaud, D. & Dreyfuss, G. (1996) Paramphistomum daubneyi: the development of redial generations in the snail Lymnaea truncatula. Parasitology Research 83, 64–69.

Aiello, S.E. (1998) The Merck veterinary manual. Whitehouse Station, New Jersey, USA, Wiley.

Anderson, P.H., Matthews, J.G., Barrett, S., Brush, P.J., Patterson, D.S. (1981). Changes in plasma enzyme activities and other blood components in response to acute and chronic liver damage in cattle. Res Vet Sci. 31: 1-4.

Andrews, S. J., & Dalton, J. P. (1999). The life cycle of Fasciola hepatica. Fasciolosis. Wallingford, UK: CABI Publishing1–29.

Arrue, E., S. Deiana and P. Muzzetto, 1970. Intestinal paramphistomiasis in ruminants; Experimental infection of sheep with metacercariae immature forms of Paramphistomum cervi. Rivista di Parassitologia, 31(1): 33-42.

Bayou K, Geda T (2018) SM Gr up SM Veterinary Medicine and Animal Science Prevalence of Bovine Fasciolosis and its Associated Risk Factors in Haranfama Municipal Abattoir, Girja District, South. 1: 1-6.

Behm, C.A. and Sangster, N.C. (1999): Pathology, pathophysiology and clinical aspects. In Dalton, J.P. (Ed.), Fasciolosis. CAB International Publishing, Wallingford, Pp. 185–224.

Bilqees, F., S. Mirza and N. Khatoon, 2011. 54. Paramphistomum Cervi Infection and Liver Tissue Damage in Buffaloes. Verlag, pp: 1-112.

Boray, J. C. (1969). "Experimental fascioliasis in Australia". Adv. Parasitolo. 7: 95–210

Bowman DD, Lynn. CR, Eberhard LM, et al. (2003) George's parasitology for veterinary.8th ed. USA: W.B. Saunders. Pp 339-347.

Bowman, Georgi, R., 2008. Georgis' Parasitology for Veterinarians (9th Ed.). W.B. Saunders Company, pp: 124.

Brown, D.S. (1980): Fresh water snails of Africa and their medical importance, Taylor and France Ltd., London. P. 487.

CDC (2012) Division of Parasitic Diseases and Malaria. (Updated 7 Nov 2012). Available at: http://www.cdc.gov/ parasites/schistosomiasis/publications.html (accessed on 07 January, 2022).

Charless. MH, Robinson. ED (2004) Diagnostic parasitology for veterinary technician 3rd ed. Chaina: Elsevier Pp 112-211.

Cheever. AW, Hoffmann. KF, Wynn. TA. (2000) Immunopathology of schistosomiasis mansoni in mice and men. Immunol Today 21:465.

Chen, M.G. and Mott, K.E. (1990): Progress in assessment of morbidity due to Fasciola *hepatica* infection: a review of recent literature. Trop. Dis. Bull. 87:1–38.

Coutinho. HM, Acosta. L.P., Wu. H.W. (2007) Th2 cytokines are associated with persistent hepatic fibrosis in human Schistosoma japonicum infection. J Infect Dis 195:288.

Dargie, J. D. (1987). The impact on production and mechanisms of pathogenesis of trematode infections in cattle and sheep. International Journal for Parasitology, 17, 453–463.

Dinnik, J.A. (1964) Intestinal paramphistomiasis and P. microbothrium Fischoeder in Africa. Bulletin of Epizootic Diseases of Africa 12, 439–454.

Dorny, P., V. Stoliaroff, J. Charlier, S. Meas, S. Sorn, B. Chea, D. Holl, D. Van Aken and J. Vercruysse, 2011. Infections with gastrointestinal nematodes, Fasciola and Paramphistomum in cattle in Cambodia and their association with morbidity parameters. Journal of Veterinary Parasitology, 175: 293-299.

Dreyfuss, G., Alarion, N., Vignoles, P., & Rondelaud, D. (2006). A retrospective study on the metacercarial production of Fasciola *hepatica* from experimentally infected Galba truncatula in central France. Parasitology Research, 98(2), 162–166.

Dube, S. and M. Aisien, 2010. Descriptive studies on Paramphistomes of small domestic ruminants in Southern Nigeria. Zimbabwe Journal of Science Technology, 5: 12-21.

Dubinský, P. (1993). Trematódy a trematodózy. PP. 158–187.

Dwight. D, Bowman. G, Georgis. M.O (2003) Parasitological for veterinarians. Elsevier (USA) pp 129-133.

Elliott, T. P., Kelley, J. M., Rawlin, G., & Spithill, T. W. (2015). High prevalence of fasciolosis and evaluation of drug efficacy against Fasciola *hepatica* in dairy cattle in the Maffra and Bairnsdale districts of Gippsland, Victoria, Australia. Veterinary Parasitology, 209(1-2), 117–124.

European Environment Agency (2004) Impacts of Europe's changing climate. An indicator-based assessment. EEA Report No. 2.

FAO (1993) The epidemiology of helminthes parasites. Available at http://www.fao.org/wairdocs/ILRI/ x5492E/x5492e04.htm-2.5%20trematodes (accessed 22 December 2021).

Fenwick. A (2012) The global burden of neglected tropical diseases. Public health 126: 233–236.

Friedman. JF, Mital. P, Kanzaria. H.K (2007) Schistosomiasis and pregnancy. Trends Parasitol 23: 159.

Fürst T, Keiser J, Utzinger J. (2012): Global burden of human food-borne trematodiasis: a systematic review and meta-analysis. Lancet Infect Dis. 12:210–21. doi: 10.1016/S1473-3099(11)70294-8

Gashaw. A (2010) Epidemiology of intestinal schistosoma in Hayk town, North East Ethiopia. Addis Ababa.

González, M., S. Lladosa, A. Castro, M. Martínez, D. Conesa, F. Munoz, A. López, Y. Manga and M. Mezo, 2013. Bovine paramphistomiasis in Galicia (Spain) prevalence, intensity, an etiology and geospatial distribution of the infection, Vetarinary Parasitology, 191: 252-263.

González, M., S. Lladosa, A. Castro, M. Martínez, D. Conesa, F. Munoz, A. López, Y. Manga and M. Mezo, 2013. Bovine paramphistomiasis in Galicia (Spain) prevalence, intensity, an etiology and geospatial distribution of the infection, Vetarinary Parasitology, 191: 252-263.

Graczyk, TK. and Fried B. (1999). "Development of Fasciola *hepatica* in the intermediate host". In: Dalton, J.P. Fasciolosis. Wallingford, Oxon, UK: CABI Pub. Pp. 31–46.

Hansen, J., & Perry, B. (1994). The epidemiology, diagnosis and control of helminth parasites of ruminants, a hand book. Nairobi, Kenya: International Laboratory for Research on Animal Disease (ILRAD).

Hendrix, C. M. and Robinson, E. (2006). Diagnostic parasitology for veterinary technicians. 3rd ed. Pp. 107 –109.

Hope-Cawdery, M. J., Strickland, K. L., Conway, A., & Crowe, P. J. (1977). Production effects of liver fluke in cattle. I. The effects of infection on live weight gain, food intake and food conversion efficiency in beef cattle. British Veterinary Journal, 133, 145–159.

http://www.dpd.cdc.gov/DPDX/HTML/Fascioliasis.htm. Life cycle of fasciola. Date of access, January 23, 2022.

https://en.wikipedia.org/w/index.php?title=Humbo&oldid=1061253685 (accessed on January 26, 2022).

Ibarra, F., Vera, Y., Quiroz, H., (2004): "Determination of the effective dose of an experimental fasciolicide in naturally and experimentally infected cattle". Vet. Parasitolo.120: 65–74.

Jacobs, D. (2009) Principles of Veterinary Parasitology 1st ed. pp330-350.

Jones, A., C. Ferreras and González, 2017. Confirmation of Galba truncatula as an intermediate host snail for Calicophoron daubneyi in Great Britain, with evidence of alternative rd snail species hosting Fasciola *hepatica*. Parasites Vectors, 8: 656.

Juyal, D., S. Kaur, Hassan and K. Paramjit, 2003. Epidemiological status of paramphistomiasis domestic ruminants in Punjab. Parasites and Diseases, 231: 235

Kogulan. P, Lucely. RD (2005) Schistosoma user medicine specialists 6: 1-11

Kowalczyk SJ, Czopowicz M, Weber CN, Müller E, Nalbert T, *et al.* (2018) Herd-level seroprevalence of Fasciola *hepatica* and Ostertagia ostertagi infection in dairy cattle population in the central and northeastern Poland. BMC Veterinary Research 1-8.

Laurent. SA, Boissier. J, Robert. A, *et al.* (2013) Schistosomiasis Chemotherapy. Angewandte Chemie (International ed. in English) 52: 7936–7956.

Lotfy, M., V. Brsant, I. Ashmawy, R. Devkota, M. Mkoji and S. Loker, 2010. A molecular approach for identification of paramphistomes from Africa and Asia. Veterinary Parasitology, 174(3-4): 234-40.

Love, S. (2017). Liver fluke- a review. Primefact 813, NSW DPI. Mage, C., Bourgne, H., Toullieu, J. M., Rondelaud, D., & Dreyfuss, G. (2002). Fasciola *hepatica* and Paramphistomum daubneyi: Changes in prevalences of natural infections in cattle and in Lymnaea truncatula from central France over the past 12 years. Veterinary Research, 33(5), 439–447.

Mandal. C.S (2012) Veterinary parasitology, 2nd ed. Kushnuma complex Basement, Ibdc publisher Pp 42-70.

Mas-Coma S, Bargues MD, Valero MA. (2005): Fascioliasis and other plant-borne trematode zoonoses. Int J Parasitol. 35:1255– 78. doi: 10.1016/j.ijpara.2005.07.010

Mas-Coma, S., Bargues, M. D., Valero, M. A. (2005): "Fascioliasis and other plant-borne trematode zoonoses". Int. J. Parasitol. 35: 1255–1278.

Melaku, S. and M. Addis, 2012. Prevalence and intensity of Paramphistomum in ruminants slaughtered at Debre Zeit industrial abattoir. Ethiopia. Global Veterinary Journal, 8(3): 315-319.

Merck. S, and Dohme. C (2010) Topic on blood parasite: The merck veterinary manual. 7th ed. USA.White house station Pp 76-78.

Mitchell, G. B., Maris, L., Bonniwell, M.A. (1998). "Triclabendazole-resistant liver fluke in Scottish sheep". Vet. Rec143: 399.

Mohammad. AA, Waqtola. C (2006) Medical Parasitology Jimma University, Ethiopia, USAID. Pp 284-300.

Moll, L., Gaasenbeek, C.P., Vellema, P., Borgsteede, F.H. (2000): "Resistance of Fasciola *hepatica* against triclabendazole in cattle and sheep in The Netherlands". Vet. Parasitol. 91: 153–158.

Njau, B. C., Kasali, O. B., Scholtens, R. G., & Mesfin, D. (1988). Review of sheep mortality in the Ethiopian highlands, 1982-1986. ILCA Bulletin, Addis Ababa, Ethiopia, 31, 19–22.

O'Brien, D.J. (1998): Fasciolosis: a threat to livestock. Iris Vet. J. 51: 539–541.

Oliveira. G, Rodrigues. NB, Romanha. AJ, *et al.* (2004) Genome and Genomics of Schistosomes.Canadian Journal of Zoology. 82: 375–390.

Olsen, O.W., 1974. Animal Parasites: Their Life Cycles and Ecology (3 ed.). Dover Publications, Inc., New York/University Park Press, Baltimore, US, pp: 273-276. ISBN 978-0486651262.

Overend, D.J., Bowen, F.L. (1995): "Resistance of Fasciola *hepatica* to triclabendazole". Aust. Vet. J. 72: 275–276.

Ozdal, N., A. Gul, F. Ilhan and S. Deger, 2010. Prevalence of Paramphistomum infection in cattle and sheep in Van Province, Turkey. Helminthologia, 47: 20-24.

Paramphistomosis in Ruminants in Ashenge, Tigray, Ethiopia Acta Parasitologica.

Piedrafita D, Spithill TW, Smith RE, Raadsma HW. (2010) Improving animal and human health through understanding liver fluke immunology. Parasite Immunol. 32:572–81. doi: 10.1111/j.1365-3024.2010. 01223.x

Qian MB, Utzinger J, Keiser J, Zhou XN. Clonorchiasis. Lancet. (2016) 387:800–10. doi: 10.1016/S0140-6736(15)60313-0

Radostits , O. M., Gay, C.C., Hinchcliff, K.W., Constable, P.D., (2007): A text book of the disease of cattle, horse, sheep, pigs and goats. 10th ed. Pp. 1576-1579.

Reinecke. RK (1997) Phylum plathlminthes veterinary helminthology, prtoria: butt heresorths Pp. 245-247, 265-273.

Rojo-Vázquez, F.A., Meana, A., Valcárcel, F. & Martínez-Valladares, M. (2012) Update on trematode infections in sheep. Veterinary Parasitology 189, 15–38.

Rolfe, F., C. Boray and H. Collins, 1994. Pathology of infection with Paramphistomum ichikawai in sheep. International Journal of Parasitology, 24: 995-1004.

Rowcliff, S.A. and Ollerenshow, C. B. (1960): Observation on the bionomics of the eggs of Fasciola *hepatica*. Ann. Trop. Med. Parasite. 54: 172 -181.

Sanabria, E. and R. Romero, 2008. "Review and update of paramphistomosis". Helminthologia, 45(2): 64-68.

Shitaye. J.E., Tsegaye. W, Paulik. I (2007) Bovine tuberculosis infection in animal and human population in Ethiopia: a review, vet. Med. 52: 332-417.

Smyth, J.D. (1994): Introduction to animal parasitology. 3rd ed. Pp.206.

Soulsby, E. J. L., (1968): Helminthes, arthropods and protozoa of domestic animals. 6th ed. Pp. 22 – 34.

Soulsby, E.J.L. (1982) Helminths, arthropods and protozoa of domesticated animals. London, Baillière Tindall.

Springer. V (2001) Taxonomic ranks under review. Available at: http://parasite.org.au/para-site/text/schistosoma-text.html.

Sykes, A.R., Coop, A.R., Robinson, M.G. (1980). Chronic subclinical ovine fascioliasis: plasma glutamate dehydrogenase, gamma glutamyl transpeptidase and aspartate aminotransferase activities and their significance as diagnostic aids. Res. Vet. Sci. 28: 71–78.

Taira, N., Yoshifuji, H., Boray, J. C. (1997): Zoonotic potential of infection with Fasciola spp. by consumption of freshly prepared raw liver containing immature flukes. Int. J. Parasitolo. 27, 775–779.

Taylor, M. A. and Coop, R. L. (2007): Veterinary Parasitology. 3rd ed. Pp. 85-89.

Thomas, A. P. (1983). The life history of the liver fluke (Fasciola *hepatica*). Quarterly J. Microscopic. Sci. 23: 99-133.

Toolan, P., K. Martinez and P. Diaz, 2015. Bovine and ovine rumen fluke in Ireland - prevalence, risk factors and species identity based on passive Veterinary surveillance and abattoir findings. Veterinary Parasitology Journal, 212: 168-174.

Torgerson, P. And Claxton, J. (1999). "Epidemiology and control." In: Dalton, J. P. Fasciolosis. Wallingford, Oxon, UK: CABI Pub. Pp. 113–49.

Tsegabirhan, K., K. Essay, H. Yohannes, W. Kidane and G. Messele, 2015. Prevalence of

Urquarhart. GM, Armour. J, Duncan. JL, *et al.* (2003) Veterinary parasitology. 2nd ed. Blackwell Sciences, scottland Pp 120-177.

Urquhart, G. M., Armour, J., Duncan, J. L., Dunn, A. M., & Jennings, F. W. (1996). Veterinary parasitology (2nd ed.). Harlow, UK: Blackwell Science Ltd102–120.

Urquhart, M., J. Armour, R. Duncan, M. Dunn and W. Len nings, 1996. Veterinary Parasitology. 2nd Ed. Longman Group Ltd., London, UK, pp: 100-109. Globalis, 6(2): 83-86.

Walz Y, Wegmann M, Dech S, Raso G, Utzinger J. (2015): Risk profiling of schistosomiasis using remote sensing: approaches, challenges and outlook. Parasit Vectors. 8:163. doi: 10.1186/s13071-015-0732-6

Yeneneh A, Kebede H, Fentahun T, Chanie M (2012) Prevalence of cattle flukes infection at Andassa Livestock Research Center in north-west of Ethiopia. Vet Res Forum 3: 85-89.

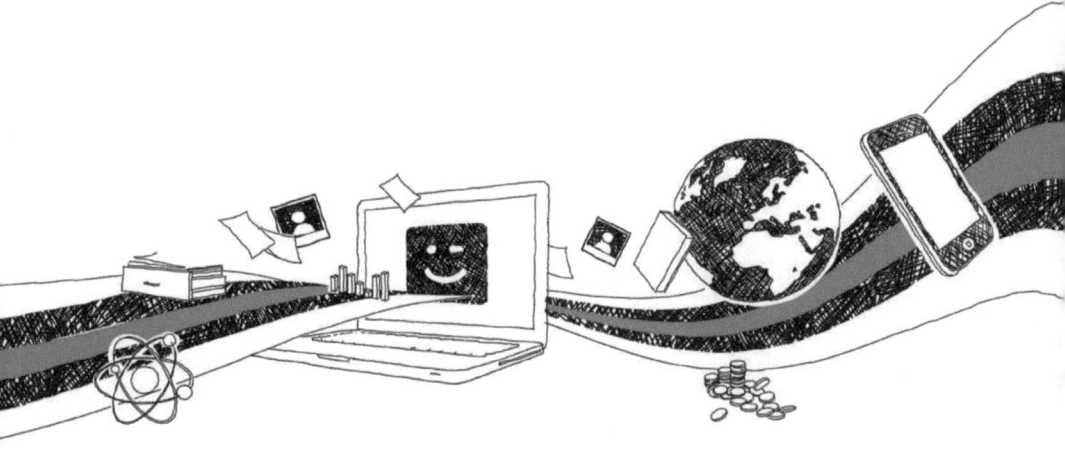
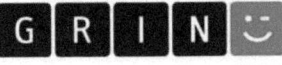